# ENDOMETRIOSIS DIET

## Nourishing Your Way to Relief and Wellness

**Dr. Raymond F. Bernard**

# TABLE OF CONTENTS

# CHAPTER 1

## Understanding Endometriosis

Endometriosis is a complex and often painful medical condition that affects millions of individuals worldwide, primarily those assigned female at birth. In this first chapter, we will delve into the world of endometriosis, providing you with a comprehensive understanding of what this condition is, its prevalence, the typical symptoms that individuals experience, and why dietary management becomes an essential aspect of coping with endometriosis.

## Introduction to Endometriosis:

Endometriosis is a chronic medical condition that occurs when tissue similar to the lining of the uterus, called endometrial tissue, grows outside the uterus. Normally, this tissue is meant to line the inside of the uterus and is shed during menstruation. However, in individuals with endometriosis, this tissue can grow on other organs in the pelvis, such as the ovaries, fallopian tubes, and the lining of the abdominal cavity. This can lead to a range of health issues and symptoms.

## Prevalence:

Endometriosis is a prevalent condition, although it is often underdiagnosed. It's estimated to affect approximately 10% of individuals of reproductive age, which translates to millions of people globally. However, because some individuals may not experience severe symptoms or may dismiss their pain as typical menstrual discomfort, many cases remain undiagnosed. This underlines the importance of raising awareness about endometriosis and the role diet can play in managing its symptoms.

## Symptoms:

Endometriosis is known for its wide range of symptoms, which can vary from person to person. Common symptoms include:

1. **Pain:** Pelvic pain is a hallmark symptom of endometriosis. This pain can occur before, during, or after menstruation and may be

severe, cramp-like, or stabbing.

2. **Heavy Menstrual Bleeding:** Endometriosis can cause heavy menstrual bleeding (menorrhagia), which can lead to anemia over time.

3. **Painful Intercourse:** Pain during sexual intercourse (dyspareunia) is another symptom that individuals with endometriosis may experience.

4. **Digestive Issues:** Endometriosis can affect the digestive system, leading to symptoms like bloating,

diarrhea, constipation, and pain during bowel movements.

5. **Infertility:** Some individuals with endometriosis may struggle with infertility, although not everyone with the condition experiences this issue.

6. **Fatigue:** The chronic pain and other symptoms of endometriosis can lead to fatigue and overall reduced quality of life.

Understanding these symptoms is crucial because they can

significantly impact an individual's physical and emotional well-being.

## The Impact of Endometriosis on Daily Life:

Endometriosis is not just about physical symptoms; it can have a profound impact on a person's daily life. The pain and discomfort associated with endometriosis can disrupt daily activities, work, and relationships. The emotional toll of living with a chronic condition can lead to anxiety, depression, and frustration.

## The Need for Dietary Management:

Given the complexity and variability of endometriosis, a multi-faceted approach to management is essential. Medications and surgical interventions are common treatment options, but diet can also play a crucial role in managing symptoms.

Dietary management is needed for several reasons:

1. **Inflammation Control:** Endometriosis is associated with chronic inflammation, and certain foods can either exacerbate or alleviate this inflammation.

Understanding which foods promote or reduce inflammation is essential for symptom management.

2. **Hormonal Balance:** Diet can influence hormonal balance in the body, particularly estrogen levels. Estrogen is known to play a key role in endometriosis, and dietary choices can impact how hormones are metabolized.

3. **Overall Health:** Eating a balanced, nutritious diet can boost overall health and immune function, helping individuals with

endometriosis better cope with the condition and its symptoms.

In this chapter, we've established the foundation for understanding endometriosis. We've explored what endometriosis is, its prevalence, the typical symptoms individuals experience, and why dietary management is crucial for those living with this condition. As we move forward in this book, we will delve deeper into the specific ways in which diet can be used as a tool to manage endometriosis and improve the quality of life for those affected.

# CHAPTER 2

## The Endometriosis-Diet Connection

In Chapter 2 of our book, "Eating for Endometriosis," we delve into the intricate relationship between diet and endometriosis. Understanding this connection is essential because it forms the basis for the dietary strategies we will explore in later chapters. Here, we explore how diet can influence the course of endometriosis, including hormonal balance and inflammation, and why this understanding is pivotal for those seeking relief from endometriosis symptoms.

## The Link Between Diet and Endometriosis:

Endometriosis is a complex condition with multiple contributing factors, and diet is one aspect that plays a significant role. It's important to recognize that diet alone cannot cure endometriosis, but it can certainly help manage its symptoms and improve overall quality of life. Let's explore two key aspects of the endometriosis-diet connection:

1. **Hormonal Balance:** One of the fundamental aspects of endometriosis is hormonal imbalance, particularly involving estrogen. Estrogen is a hormone that influences the growth and behavior of endometrial tissue. Diet plays a role in hormonal balance because certain foods contain compounds that can either mimic or modulate estrogen in the body.

2. **Inflammation Control:** Chronic inflammation is another hallmark of

endometriosis. The immune system's response to endometrial tissue outside the uterus triggers inflammation, leading to pain and other symptoms. Diet can influence the body's inflammatory response, either exacerbating or reducing inflammation.

**Estrogen and Diet:**

Estrogen dominance is often observed in individuals with endometriosis, meaning they have higher levels of estrogen relative to progesterone. This imbalance can contribute to the growth and spread of endometrial tissue outside the uterus. Dietary choices can impact estrogen levels in several ways:

- **Phytoestrogens:** Some plant-based foods contain compounds called phytoestrogens that can weakly mimic estrogen in the body. These include foods like soy, flaxseeds, and legumes. In some cases, incorporating moderate amounts of these foods may help balance estrogen levels.
- **Fiber:** Dietary fiber, found in fruits, vegetables, and

whole grains, aids in estrogen metabolism. It helps the body excrete excess estrogen, preventing its buildup. This is why a high-fiber diet can be beneficial for individuals with endometriosis.

- **Protein Sources:** Different protein sources, such as animal and plant-based proteins, can have varying effects on estrogen levels. For instance, diets high in red meat have been associated with higher estrogen levels, while plant-based diets may have the opposite effect.

**Inflammation and Diet:**

Chronic inflammation is a key driver of pain and discomfort in endometriosis. Diet plays a pivotal role in either promoting or reducing inflammation. Here's how:

- **Omega-3 Fatty Acids:** Foods rich in omega-3 fatty acids, such as fatty fish, flaxseeds, and walnuts, possess anti-inflammatory properties. They can help reduce inflammation, potentially alleviating endometriosis-related pain.

- **Antioxidants:** Fruits and vegetables, particularly those with vibrant colors like berries, contain antioxidants that combat oxidative stress and inflammation. Including these foods in your diet can be beneficial.

- **Pro-Inflammatory Foods:** On the flip side, certain foods can promote inflammation. These include processed foods, sugary snacks, and trans fats. Limiting the consumption of these items can help manage inflammation.

Understanding how diet influences hormones and inflammation is the first step toward using food as a tool to manage endometriosis symptoms. It's important to emphasize that the impact of diet can vary from person to person. What works for one individual may not work for another, and that's why personalized dietary approaches are often recommended.

In this chapter, we've laid the foundation for the critical connection between diet and endometriosis. By recognizing how diet can influence hormonal balance and inflammation, individuals with endometriosis can make informed dietary choices. In subsequent chapters, we'll dive deeper into specific dietary strategies, including foods to include and avoid, to help you manage your endometriosis symptoms effectively.

# CHAPTER 3

## Building a Foundation: Nutritional Basics

In Chapter 3 of our book, "Eating for Endometriosis," we embark on a journey through the essential nutritional principles that form the foundation for managing endometriosis symptoms through diet. Understanding these nutritional basics is crucial because they provide the framework upon which you can develop a dietary plan tailored to your unique needs.

## The Importance of a Balanced Diet:

Maintaining a balanced diet is key for overall health and is especially important when you're dealing with a chronic condition like endometriosis. A balanced diet ensures that you're getting all the essential nutrients your body needs to function optimally. Here are some key aspects of a balanced diet:

- **Macronutrients:** A balanced diet includes the right balance of macronutrients: carbohydrates, proteins, and fats. Carbohydrates provide energy, proteins repair and build tissues, and fats are essential for many bodily functions.

- **Micronutrients:** In addition to macronutrients, a balanced diet should also provide essential micronutrients, such as vitamins and minerals. These nutrients play vital roles in various bodily processes, from maintaining a strong immune system to supporting bone health.

- **Fiber:** Dietary fiber, found in fruits, vegetables, whole grains, and legumes, is crucial for digestive health. It also helps regulate blood sugar levels and may assist in managing endometriosis-related inflammation.

- **Hydration:** Staying well-hydrated is essential for overall health. Water supports digestion, regulates body temperature, and helps transport nutrients throughout the body.

## Key Nutrients for Managing Endometriosis:

While a balanced diet is essential, certain nutrients deserve special attention when managing endometriosis symptoms:

- **Omega-3 Fatty Acids:** These are powerful anti-inflammatory nutrients found in fatty fish like salmon, walnuts, flaxseeds, and chia seeds. Including these foods in your diet may help reduce inflammation associated with endometriosis.

- **Iron:** Heavy menstrual bleeding is a common symptom of endometriosis and can lead to iron deficiency anemia.

Incorporating iron-rich foods like lean meats, beans, lentils, and leafy greens can help prevent or alleviate anemia.

- **Calcium and Vitamin D:** Some individuals with endometriosis may be at risk of reduced bone density, especially if they've been on long-term hormonal treatments. Calcium-rich foods like dairy products or fortified plant-based alternatives and vitamin D from sunlight exposure or supplements can support bone health.

- **Folate:** Folate, found in leafy greens, citrus fruits, and legumes, is important for cell repair and function. It's also beneficial for managing endometriosis-related inflammation.

- **Magnesium:** This mineral plays a role in muscle and nerve function and can help alleviate muscle cramps and pain associated with endometriosis. Magnesium-rich foods include nuts, seeds, and whole grains.

## Portion Control and Meal Planning:

Maintaining the right portion sizes and planning your meals effectively can make a significant difference in managing endometriosis symptoms:

- **Balancing Your Plate:** A well-balanced meal typically includes a source of lean protein, whole grains, plenty of vegetables, and a small amount of healthy fats. This combination helps stabilize blood sugar levels and provides a range of nutrients.

- **Meal Frequency:** Eating smaller, balanced meals

more frequently throughout the day can help stabilize energy levels and manage hunger. This can be especially beneficial for those with endometriosis who may experience fluctuations in appetite.

- **Mindful Eating:** Paying attention to your body's hunger and fullness cues is essential. Eating slowly and savoring your food can help prevent overeating and improve digestion.

- **Meal Prep:** Planning your meals and snacks in advance can make it easier to stick to a balanced diet. It also reduces the temptation to reach for unhealthy convenience foods.

By focusing on these nutritional basics, you're laying the groundwork for a diet that supports your overall health and specifically addresses some of the challenges posed by endometriosis. In the following chapters, we'll build upon this foundation by exploring specific foods to include and avoid, as well as diving deeper into the role of nutrition in managing endometriosis-related

inflammation and hormonal
balance.

# CHAPTER 4

## Foods to Include

In Chapter 4 of our book, "Eating for Endometriosis," we delve into a critical aspect of managing endometriosis through diet - the selection of foods to include in your daily meals. These are foods that can aid in symptom relief, promote hormonal balance, and reduce inflammation, all of which are essential for effectively managing endometriosis.

## Anti-Inflammatory Foods and Their Benefits:

Chronic inflammation is a significant contributor to the pain and discomfort associated with endometriosis. Therefore, incorporating anti-inflammatory foods into your diet can be highly beneficial. Here are some key categories of anti-inflammatory foods and their benefits:

- **Fruits and Vegetables:** These are packed with antioxidants, vitamins, and minerals. The vibrant colors of fruits and vegetables often indicate the presence of anti-inflammatory compounds. For instance, berries are rich in anthocyanins, which have potent anti-inflammatory properties.

- **Fatty Fish:** Salmon, mackerel, sardines, and other fatty fish are excellent sources of omega-3 fatty acids. These healthy fats have been shown to reduce inflammation and may help alleviate endometriosis-related pain.

- **Nuts and Seeds:** Almonds, walnuts, flaxseeds, and chia seeds are high in healthy fats, fiber, and antioxidants.

They can be great additions to your diet to combat inflammation.

- **Whole Grains:** Whole grains like oats, brown rice, and quinoa provide complex carbohydrates and fiber, which can help stabilize blood sugar levels and reduce inflammation.

- **Herbs and Spices:** Turmeric, ginger, and garlic are well-known for their anti-inflammatory properties. These can be used as seasonings in your cooking to add flavor and reduce inflammation.

**Nutrient-Rich Foods for Symptom Relief:**

Endometriosis often comes with a range of symptoms, including pain, heavy bleeding, and digestive issues. Certain nutrient-rich foods can help alleviate these symptoms:

- **Iron-Rich Foods:** If you experience heavy menstrual bleeding, replenishing iron stores is essential. Lean meats, beans, lentils, and dark leafy greens like spinach and kale are excellent sources of iron.
- **Fiber-Rich Foods:** Fiber can help regulate bowel

movements and reduce bloating, which is especially beneficial if you have digestive issues. Whole grains, fruits, vegetables, and legumes are all high in fiber.

- **Calcium and Vitamin D Sources:** To support bone health, especially if you're on long-term hormonal treatments, consider dairy products or fortified plant-based alternatives for calcium and get adequate sunlight exposure or take vitamin D supplements.

- **Folate and B Vitamins:** These nutrients support overall health and can help manage inflammation. You can find them in leafy greens, citrus fruits, and whole grains.

- **Lean Proteins:** Lean sources of protein, such as poultry, fish, tofu, and legumes, are vital for muscle repair and overall health.

## Recipes and Meal Ideas:

To make incorporating these foods into your diet easier, we provide you with a selection of delicious recipes and meal ideas in this chapter. These recipes are carefully crafted to include ingredients that are not only nutritious but also flavorful and satisfying. Here are a few examples:

- **Berry and Spinach Smoothie:** Blend spinach, frozen berries, a banana, Greek yogurt (or a dairy-free alternative), and a tablespoon of flaxseeds for a nutrient-packed breakfast or snack.

- **Salmon with Quinoa and Roasted Vegetables:** Season a salmon fillet with herbs and bake it alongside a mixture of your favorite vegetables and cooked quinoa for a balanced and anti-inflammatory dinner.

- **Chickpea and Vegetable Curry:** Make a hearty, plant-based curry with chickpeas, plenty of vegetables, and a flavorful blend of spices like turmeric, cumin, and coriander.

- **Avocado and Walnut Salad:** Combine ripe avocado, walnuts, mixed greens, cherry tomatoes, and a drizzle of olive oil for a nutrient-dense salad.

By incorporating these foods and recipes into your diet, you can take a proactive approach to managing endometriosis symptoms. Remember that it's not just about what you eat but also how you prepare and enjoy your meals. Eating mindfully and savoring the flavors can enhance your overall dining experience.

This chapter serves as a practical guide to help you make informed dietary choices that align with your goal of managing endometriosis. In the following chapters, we'll explore the other side of the coin - foods to avoid -

and provide you with strategies to create balanced and endometriosis-friendly meal plans.

# CHAPTER 5

## Foods to Avoid

In Chapter 5 of our book, "Eating for Endometriosis," we dive into the critical topic of foods to avoid. Understanding which foods can potentially worsen endometriosis symptoms is just as important as knowing which foods can help manage them. This chapter explores dietary triggers that can exacerbate inflammation, hormonal imbalances, and discomfort associated with endometriosis.

# Trigger Foods and Endometriosis:

Endometriosis is a condition characterized by inflammation and hormonal imbalance, and certain foods can contribute to these issues. Here, we identify common trigger foods and explain how they can negatively impact endometriosis:

1. **Dairy Products:** Dairy is a source of saturated fats and can contain hormones and growth factors that might exacerbate hormonal imbalances in individuals with endometriosis. Some

people also have lactose intolerance, which can lead to digestive issues.

2. **Red Meat:** Red meat, particularly processed meats like sausages and bacon, is high in saturated fats, which can promote inflammation. Additionally, some red meats may contain hormones and antibiotics.

3. **Gluten-Containing Grains:** For some individuals with endometriosis, gluten can trigger digestive issues and inflammation. Wheat,

barley, and rye are common sources of gluten.

4. **Caffeine:** Caffeine, found in coffee, tea, and many soft drinks, can irritate the gastrointestinal tract and exacerbate symptoms like bloating and cramps.

5. **Alcohol:** Alcohol can disrupt hormonal balance, contribute to inflammation, and affect liver function, which plays a role in metabolizing hormones.

6. **Sugary Foods:** High-sugar foods and drinks can lead to blood sugar spikes and crashes, potentially

worsening inflammation and pain.

7. **Highly Processed Foods:** Foods high in trans fats, artificial additives, and preservatives can contribute to inflammation and digestive discomfort.

## Strategies for Reducing Dietary Triggers:

While these trigger foods can exacerbate endometriosis symptoms for some individuals, it's essential to remember that dietary sensitivities vary from person to person. What triggers symptoms in one person may not affect another. Here are some strategies for identifying and reducing dietary triggers:

1. **Food Diary:** Keeping a food diary can help you track your diet and symptoms over time, enabling you to pinpoint specific trigger foods.

2. **Elimination Diet:** Under the guidance of a healthcare professional or dietitian, you can embark on an elimination diet to systematically remove potential trigger foods and

gradually reintroduce them
to gauge their impact.

3. **Personalized Approach:**
Remember that individual
responses to foods vary.
What may be a trigger for
one person might not be an
issue for another. It's crucial
to tailor your diet based on
your specific symptoms and
sensitivities.

4. **Gradual Changes:** Making
dietary changes gradually
can make the process more
manageable and help you
identify specific triggers
more effectively.

5. **Alternative Choices:** When eliminating trigger foods, seek out alternative choices that align with your dietary needs and preferences. For example, if dairy is a trigger, explore dairy-free milk alternatives like almond, soy, or oat milk.

## Balanced Eating Despite Restrictions:

Eliminating trigger foods doesn't mean you have to compromise a balanced diet. You can still enjoy a variety of nutrient-rich foods that support your health and manage endometriosis. Here's how:

- **Diversify Your Plate:** Focus on a colorful array of fruits and vegetables, lean proteins, and whole grains that align with your dietary restrictions.

- **Experiment with Alternative Ingredients:** Explore gluten-free grains like quinoa, amaranth, or rice, and try plant-based protein sources like tofu, tempeh, or legumes if you've cut back on red meat.

- **Cook at Home:** Preparing meals at home allows you to have full control over the ingredients you use, making it easier to avoid trigger foods.

- **Seek Professional Guidance:** If you're concerned about nutritional deficiencies due to dietary restrictions, consider consulting with a registered dietitian who can help you create a well-balanced meal plan.

Chapter 5 provides you with the knowledge and tools you need to identify and avoid trigger foods that may worsen your endometriosis symptoms. By taking a personalized approach to your diet and gradually making adjustments, you can work toward a diet that supports your health and reduces discomfort. In the following chapters, we'll delve further into specific dietary strategies, including those that focus on hormone balance and inflammation control.

# CHAPTER 6

## Hormone-Balancing Diet

In Chapter 6 of our book, "Eating for Endometriosis," we delve into the intricate relationship between diet and hormonal balance. Hormones, especially estrogen, play a significant role in endometriosis, and understanding how your diet can influence hormone levels is crucial for effectively managing your symptoms.

**Estrogen and Endometriosis:**

Estrogen is a sex hormone that plays a central role in the development and progression of endometriosis. This hormone promotes the growth of endometrial tissue, which can lead to the formation of painful lesions outside the uterus. For individuals with endometriosis, it's often essential to address estrogen dominance, which occurs when there's an excess of estrogen relative to progesterone.

## Dietary Factors Influencing Estrogen Levels:

Several dietary factors can influence estrogen levels in the body, which is why a hormone-balancing diet is a valuable tool in managing endometriosis:

1. **Phytoestrogens:** Some plant-based foods contain compounds called phytoestrogens, which can mimic or modulate estrogen in the body. These include soy products, flaxseeds, sesame seeds, and legumes. While phytoestrogens can be beneficial for some individuals by balancing estrogen levels, they should be consumed in moderation,

especially if estrogen dominance is a concern.

2. **Fiber:** Dietary fiber, found in fruits, vegetables, and whole grains, plays a vital role in hormone metabolism. It helps the body excrete excess estrogen, reducing its accumulation in the body.

3. **Healthy Fats:** Consuming healthy fats, such as those found in fatty fish (rich in omega-3 fatty acids), avocados, nuts, and seeds, can support hormone balance. These fats aid in the production of hormones and

can help reduce inflammation.

## Hormone-Balancing Foods and Herbs:

In this chapter, we explore specific foods and herbs that can promote hormonal balance and alleviate endometriosis symptoms:

1. **Cruciferous Vegetables:** Foods like broccoli, cauliflower, Brussels sprouts, and kale contain compounds that support liver function, helping the body metabolize estrogen more efficiently.

2. **Herbal Teas:** Some herbal teas, such as spearmint and chamomile, have been associated with hormonal balance and reduced menstrual pain. These teas can be soothing and beneficial additions to your diet.

3. **Omega-3 Fatty Acids:** As mentioned earlier, omega-3-rich foods like fatty fish, flaxseeds, and walnuts can help reduce inflammation and support hormonal balance.

4. **Vitex (Chasteberry):** This herbal remedy is known for

its potential to regulate the menstrual cycle and balance hormones. It's available in supplement form but should be used under the guidance of a healthcare professional.

**Balancing Hormones with Food:**

A hormone-balancing diet involves making conscious choices about the foods you consume to promote hormonal harmony. Here are some dietary strategies to consider:

- **Moderate Phytoestrogens:** If

estrogen dominance is a concern, moderate your intake of phytoestrogen-rich foods. Pay attention to how your body responds and adjust your diet accordingly.

- **Fiber-Rich Diet:** Prioritize a high-fiber diet to support estrogen excretion. Incorporate a variety of fruits, vegetables, and whole grains into your meals.

- **Healthy Fats:** Include sources of healthy fats like avocados, olive oil, and fatty fish in your diet to support hormone production and reduce inflammation.

- **Hydration:** Staying well-hydrated is essential for hormone balance. Water helps transport hormones throughout the body and supports their function.

- **Portion Control:** Maintain balanced portion sizes to manage calorie intake and prevent weight gain, which can influence hormone balance.

- **Consult a Healthcare Professional:** If you're considering herbal supplements or significant dietary changes to address hormonal imbalances, consult with a healthcare provider or a registered dietitian. They can provide personalized guidance tailored to your specific needs.

## The Hormone-Balancing Diet in Practice:

This chapter goes beyond theory and provides practical guidance on how to incorporate hormone-balancing foods and herbs into your daily meals. It offers recipes and meal plans that focus on supporting hormonal harmony and reducing the impact of endometriosis on your life.

Understanding how your diet can influence hormone balance is a vital component of managing endometriosis. By adopting a hormone-balancing diet and making informed dietary choices, you can potentially alleviate symptoms and improve your overall quality of life. In the following chapters, we'll continue to explore holistic dietary strategies for managing endometriosis, including inflammation control and long-term lifestyle changes.

# CHAPTER 7

## Supplements and Herbs

In Chapter 7 of our book, "Eating for Endometriosis," we delve into the world of supplements and herbal remedies as complementary approaches to managing endometriosis. While a well-balanced diet is crucial, supplements and herbs can be valuable additions to your regimen, offering potential benefits in symptom relief, hormone regulation, and inflammation control.

## The Role of Supplements in Endometriosis Management:

Supplements are concentrated forms of specific nutrients that can be used to address nutritional deficiencies, support overall health, and manage specific symptoms related to endometriosis.

**1. Omega-3 Fatty Acids:** Omega-3 supplements, such as fish oil capsules or vegan alternatives like algae oil, provide a concentrated source of these anti-inflammatory fats. Omega-3s have shown promise in reducing inflammation, potentially alleviating endometriosis-related pain and discomfort. It's important to choose a high-quality supplement and consult with a healthcare provider for appropriate dosing.

**2. Iron:** Iron supplements may be necessary if you have iron-deficiency anemia due to heavy menstrual bleeding. They can help restore your iron levels and reduce fatigue. Always consult with a healthcare professional before starting iron supplementation to determine the right dosage and form for your needs.

**3. Vitamin D:** Many people with endometriosis have been found to have lower vitamin D levels. Vitamin D is essential for bone health and immune function. Your healthcare provider may recommend vitamin D supplements to address deficiencies. However, it's important to monitor your vitamin D levels and adjust supplementation accordingly.

**4. Calcium:** If you've reduced your dairy intake due to dietary sensitivities or preferences, calcium supplements or fortified plant-based milk alternatives can help you meet your calcium needs. Adequate calcium intake supports bone health, especially important if you're on long-term hormonal treatments.

## Herbal Remedies and Their Potential Benefits:

Herbs have been used for centuries in traditional medicine to manage various health conditions, including those related to menstruation and pelvic pain. While the scientific evidence regarding herbal remedies for endometriosis is limited, some herbs have shown promise in managing symptoms.

**1. Vitex (Chasteberry):** Vitex is a popular herbal remedy believed to help regulate the menstrual cycle and balance hormones. It may be particularly beneficial for individuals with irregular periods or hormonal imbalances. It's available in various forms, including capsules and tinctures, but should be used under the guidance of a healthcare professional.

**2. Turmeric:** Turmeric contains an active compound called curcumin, known for its anti-inflammatory properties. While more research is needed, some individuals with endometriosis have reported reduced pain and inflammation with turmeric supplementation. You can find curcumin supplements or incorporate turmeric into your diet.

**3. Ginger:** Ginger has anti-inflammatory and pain-relieving properties and may provide relief from endometriosis-related pain and digestive discomfort. You can consume ginger as a supplement, in tea, or by adding it to your meals.

**4. Evening Primrose Oil:** Evening primrose oil contains

gamma-linolenic acid (GLA), a type of omega-6 fatty acid. Some women with endometriosis have reported symptom relief with GLA supplements. Consult with a healthcare provider for appropriate dosing.

**Safety and Considerations:**

While supplements and herbs can offer potential benefits, it's crucial to approach them with caution:

- Always consult with a healthcare provider before starting any new supplement or herbal remedy, especially if you have underlying health conditions or are taking medications.

- Be mindful of potential interactions between supplements, herbs, and medications you may be using.

- Purchase supplements from reputable sources to ensure quality and purity.

- Start with the lowest effective dose and monitor your response.

- Supplements and herbs are not a replacement for a well-balanced diet. They should complement your dietary efforts rather than serve as a primary solution.

## Holistic Approach to Endometriosis Management:

Chapter 7 emphasizes the importance of a holistic approach to endometriosis management. Supplements and herbs can be valuable tools when used in conjunction with dietary changes, lifestyle modifications, and any medical treatments prescribed by your healthcare provider.

Remember that individual responses to supplements and herbs vary. What works for one person may not work for another, so it's essential to adopt a personalized approach to your endometriosis management plan. A healthcare provider or a registered herbalist can provide guidance tailored to your specific needs.

In the final chapter of our book, we'll tie together all the elements discussed so far, offering strategies for long-term management and sustainable dietary choices to support your journey toward better health and symptom relief in the context of endometriosis.

# CHAPTER 8

## Sustainable Endometriosis Management

In the final chapter of our book, "Eating for Endometriosis," we address the importance of long-term, sustainable management strategies. Endometriosis is a chronic condition, and while dietary changes and complementary approaches can offer significant relief, a consistent and holistic approach is key to effectively managing the condition over time.

1. **The Power of Consistency:** Consistency is the cornerstone of managing endometriosis effectively. It's not just about making short-term dietary changes or using supplements for a brief period. Sustainable management involves integrating these changes into your daily life.

2. **Building Healthy Habits:** Building healthy habits is essential for long-term success. These habits may include regular exercise, stress management techniques, and getting enough

sleep. When combined with a balanced diet, these habits can help reduce inflammation, manage pain, and improve overall well-being.

3. **Mindful Eating:** Mindful eating involves being present and fully engaged with your meals. Pay attention to your body's hunger and fullness cues, savor the flavors of your food, and eat with intention. This practice can help prevent overeating and promote better digestion.

4. **Regular Monitoring:** Monitoring your symptoms and how they relate to your diet and

lifestyle is crucial. Keep a journal to track your menstrual cycle, pain levels, and dietary choices. This can help you identify patterns and make informed adjustments.

5. **Adapting as Needed:** As your body changes and responds to various management strategies, be willing to adapt your approach. What worked for you in the past may not work forever. Consulting with healthcare providers or nutrition experts periodically can help you fine-tune your plan.

6. **Managing Stress:** Chronic stress can exacerbate endometriosis symptoms.

Incorporate stress management techniques such as meditation, deep breathing exercises, yoga, or hobbies that relax you into your daily routine.

7. **Community and Support:** Joining a support group or seeking the support of friends and family can be invaluable. Sharing your experiences, challenges, and successes with others who understand what you're going through can provide emotional and practical support.

8. **Advocating for Yourself:** Be an advocate for your own health. Keep up-to-date with the latest

research and treatment options for endometriosis. If your symptoms persist or worsen, don't hesitate to seek further medical advice and treatment.

9. **Holistic Approach:** Recognize that endometriosis management isn't just about diet or supplements alone. It's about adopting a holistic approach that addresses all aspects of your health, including physical, emotional, and mental well-being.

10. **Educating Others:** Endometriosis is a condition that often goes misunderstood. Educating friends, family, and

colleagues about your condition can help create a supportive environment and reduce stigma.

**Celebrating Progress:** Along your journey, remember to celebrate your progress, no matter how small it may seem. Managing endometriosis is a long-term endeavor, and acknowledging your achievements can provide motivation and a sense of accomplishment.

**Setting Realistic Expectations:** Managing endometriosis is not about finding a one-size-fits-all solution. It's about finding what works for you and adapting as needed. Understand that there may be good days and challenging days, but with consistent effort and the right support, you can enhance your quality of life.

**Seeking Professional Guidance:** As you navigate your endometriosis management journey, consider seeking guidance from healthcare providers, including gynecologists, dietitians, and mental health professionals. They can offer tailored advice and support based on your unique needs.

## Conclusion: A Lifelong Journey

In the concluding chapter, we emphasize that managing endometriosis is a lifelong journey. While dietary changes and complementary approaches are powerful tools, they are part of a broader strategy that includes adopting healthy habits, managing stress, and seeking professional guidance when necessary. With dedication, patience, and a holistic approach, individuals with endometriosis can enhance their quality of life and work towards better symptom management.

This book has provided you with a comprehensive understanding of endometriosis, its impact on your health, and how diet and lifestyle changes can help alleviate symptoms. It has equipped you with knowledge about foods to include and avoid, the role of nutrition in hormonal balance and inflammation control, and the potential benefits of supplements and herbs.

As you continue on your journey to manage endometriosis, remember that you are not alone. Seek support from healthcare providers, support groups, and loved ones. Be adaptable and open to changes in your approach, and above all, prioritize self-care and self-compassion. By doing so, you can take charge of your health and lead a fulfilling life despite the challenges of endometriosis.

# CONCLUSION

## Empowering Your Journey with Endometriosis

In the pages of "Eating for Endometriosis," we have embarked on a journey of empowerment and discovery. This book has been crafted to provide you with the knowledge, tools, and strategies needed to navigate the complex landscape of endometriosis with resilience and hope.

Endometriosis is a challenging condition, one that can often leave individuals feeling powerless and overwhelmed. Yet, within these pages, we've illuminated a path toward taking control of your health and well-being. It's a path defined by informed choices, nourishing foods, mindful practices, and a holistic approach to managing the various facets of your life impacted by this condition.

From understanding the intricate relationship between diet, hormones, and inflammation to identifying trigger foods and incorporating nourishing alternatives, we've equipped you with the essentials for crafting a personalized dietary plan that aligns with your unique needs. We've explored the potential benefits of supplements and herbs, providing you with insights into how these natural remedies can complement your journey toward relief and healing.

However, this book goes beyond the realm of food. It recognizes that managing endometriosis is a holistic endeavor, one that encompasses physical, emotional, and mental well-being. It encourages you to embrace sustainable habits, to manage stress, to build a support network, and to advocate for yourself in the realm of healthcare.

Above all, this book is an affirmation of your resilience and strength. It's a reminder that while endometriosis may be a part of your life, it does not define you. You have the power to shape your path, to celebrate your successes, and to navigate the challenges with courage and grace.

As you continue your journey with endometriosis, know that you are not alone. Millions of individuals around the world face similar battles, and there is a community of support waiting to embrace you.

Seek guidance when needed, share your experiences, and remember to celebrate each step forward, no matter how small it may seem.

In closing, "Eating for Endometriosis" is more than just a book; it is a testament to your strength, your resilience, and your capacity for growth. May the knowledge and insights within these pages empower you to live a life filled with vitality and hope, no matter the challenges that may come your way. You are not alone on this journey, and your path is one of courage and empowerment.

www.ingramcontent.com/pod-product-compliance
Lightning Source LLC
Chambersburg PA
CBHW050738260726

48661CB00001B/303